Axcio

MW01268823

The Complete Guide to Quick Weight Loss and Ending Obesity

Nancy Bond

Acxion Fentermina

Acxion is a solution pill for weight decrease. Phentermine is the main ingredient in Acxion. The Acxion pill's main goal is to suppress appetite, which means people eat less and always lose too much weight. A Mexican pharmaceutical company is responsible for the production of Acxion.

Acxion is medications that help people who are obese lose weight. It works through method of method for animating the nerve center, which is in expense of feeling hungry, and subsequently, the desire for food is decreased. These pills are designed to assist you in losing weight. It is a marked variant of the pharmacological hunger suppressant Phentermine, what imparts substance properties to amphetamines. Acxion is a weight loss supplement that can only be purchased online through.

Acxion is used to measure fatness if your body mass index is 30 or higher. The pill can be taken if you are overweight and have a body mass index greater than 30. If you have type 2 diabetes or arterial hypertension and your weight is steadily rising, you can also take this pill.

Common Problems with Men Losing Weight

One of the main concerns men have about losing weight is how realistically they approach dieting. While numerous men might demand that they are having exercise meetings every day, this doesn't basically mean they are losing their extreme weight; in point of fact, they will tone up. As men get older, healthy eating and exercise can sometimes make it hard for them to lose weight.

Despite this, it is common knowledge that most men can lose two to five kilograms in a week. It would be more harmful and have serious side effects if anyone wanted to lose weight faster. However, as obesity rates rise, weight loss has emerged as a major issue. It is essential to emphasize that weight gain can be caused by a variety of factors, regardless of whether you are naturally inclined to do so, which is debatable; whether you have enormous bones; or then again whether you just put on weight more oftentimes than your kin or other relatives. These factors may include how much you eat, the kinds of foods you eat, and whether you are active or sedentary.

The amount of weight lost depends on a number of health factors, which can only be checked by your doctor. Men are in a better position to lose weight as they get older because the issues they have with their weight begin to come to light. If you're overweight, you should follow a healthy diet and exercise every day to stay fit and live a healthy life. You don't have to take undesirable bites and all of the greasy broiled and awful food varieties you have been appreciating while at the same time eating them. You simply have to eat lean meats and less greasy items that convey fiber and supplements to your body that might be deficient in your eating routine.

Weight loss pills made of natural ingredients are few and far between. These pills cut down your body fats and lessen unnecessary weight. Your caloric intake will be reduced to a manageable level as a result of these pills having a direct effect on your brain. What's more, this impact will at last assist you with lessening the unnecessary load of your body. [Text Wrapping Break]These Acxion pills are clinically proven and have more advanced results. Acxion Fentermina is the safest and best weight loss pill.

What is Acxion?

Weight loss medication Acxion is prescribed. Phentermine is the main ingredient in Acxion. The Acxion pill's main goal is to suppress appetite, which means people eat less and always lose too much weight. A Mexican pharmaceutical company is responsible for the production of Acxion.

These pills were made to help people who were overweight lose weight. Acxion pills have the ability to stimulate the central nervous system, resulting in an increase in heart rate, blood pressure, and appetite. As a result, you will feel less hungry and eat less food. Obesity is treated with this pill, along with diet and exercise, especially in people who have high risk factors like diabetes, high blood pressure, or cholesterol.

This is a diet pill that suppresses your appetite and helps you lose weight. It also helps you get rid of extra fat from your body. Phentermine-based Acxion pills claim to help people lose weight by controlling how the central nervous system works to help them resist food cravings. However, in contrast to other weight loss supplements, this one requires a prescription and is only prescribed if the individual has been diagnosed as being medically overweight and has medical reasons to lose weight.

Ingredients in Acxion:

These pills contain numerous ingredients, but Phentermine—the only active ingredient—is the primary ingredient. These pills likewise have phentermine hydrochloride in them. These pills are available in two specific dosages: 15 milligrams for immediate release and 30 milligrams for extended release.

How does Phentermine work?

Phentermine is similar to amphetamine, a prescription drug used to suppress appetite, in that it is a chemical intoxicant. By making you feel fuller for longer or decreasing your hunger, this pill can help you lose weight. These pills are likewise accessible in blend with topiramate for weight decrease.

Phentermine positively adjusts certain body functions by stimulating the central nervous system. It is because of this that it is also known to suppress appetite.

How Does Acxion Function?

Phentermine, the primary ingredient in Acxion, is a member of the anorectic (also known as hunger suppressant) class of pills. [Text Wrapping Break]Acxion Fentermine helps you get rid of the symptoms of obsessive overeating by suppressing your appetite. As a result, you will eat fewer calories, which will help you lose weight. Other eating disorders can also be treated with these pills. Topiramate is combined with the pill to increase the effect. Researchers say that overeating is made possible by an increase in brain levels of neurotransmitters. We advise only purchasing Acxion from the company's official website.

This is the same way Acxion Fentermina makes you feel less hungry: it makes your brain produce more neurotransmitters in response. Your body's chemical messengers are neurotransmitters. When your body has higher levels of these chemicals, you feel less compelled to eat, which makes you lose weight. Due to the effects of phentermine, your body will develop a tolerance to hunger if you take these pills for a few weeks.

By paying close attention to your diet and adding exercise to your daily routine. This impact will ultimately assist you with decreasing generally speaking body overabundance weight.

How to Utilize Acxion?

This pill might be utilized orally as coordinated by your PCP, frequently once day to day, one hour preceding breakfast or one to two hours after breakfast. Your doctor can make any necessary dosage adjustments based on your body condition. To diminish incidental effects however much as could reasonably be expected, kindly adhere to your PCP's directions. On the off chance that you take these pills late in the day, this might create problems dozing.

The endorsed sum and time period depend on your body's ailment and its reaction to treatment. Your doctor will adjust the dose according to what works best for you. You can go through the benefits and inconveniences, as well as the time between Acxion medicines, with your primary care physician. To get the best results, take this medication as directed, on a regular basis, and for the full time prescribed by your doctor.

By checking your body, your doctor can prescribe taking the pill as part of a short-term, several-week, or long-term course. Additionally, it is recommended that you avoid overeating and incorporate physical activity into your routine.

If you stop taking this medication suddenly, you may experience symptoms like severe tiredness and depression. Your doctor will gradually lower your dosage to help prevent symptoms.

After a few weeks of use, taking this medication in excess may stop working as intended. Talk to your doctor if this medication suddenly stops working well for you. Except if your PCP teaches you to do as such, never support the measurement all alone. By examining your body, your doctor may permit you to stop taking this medication.

How to Take Acxion Pills?

Typically, Acxion pills come in three strengths: 6.4 mg, 15 mg, and 30 mg. Therefore, one can take these pills in one of the following ways:

Acxion Fentermina 6.4mg (multiple times day to day)

Acxion Fentermina 15mg (twice day to day)

Acxion Fentermina 30mg (when day to day)

Notwithstanding, to forestall unfavorable impacts, the everyday most extreme portion of Acxion is 30mg.

Common Side Effects Following Acxion use, your body may experience the following side effects:

Dry mouth and an unpleasant taste in the mouth are common side effects of Acxion pills. In case of an excess, you may likewise encounter gastrointestinal issues like tooting, the runs, or clogging.

When you take these pills, you might feel sick, and in rare cases, you might vomit. You may feel something in your chest while taking a pill to heal you.

Unwanted reactions to these pills may occur in your central nervous system. You also have the option of expressing your severe and unnecessary worry as well as your agitation, which can occur in the morning as well as in the afternoon. As a result, you might feel helpless and scared.

These medications cause insomnia in the majority of women. This is thought to cause difficulty falling asleep and frequent nighttime awakenings.

You can awaken in light of the fact that you have bad dreams as the symptoms of these pills.

Additionally, you may experience an allergic reaction, which typically manifests as a small, itchy rash on your skin following the administration of Acxion tablets. Just the people who have a background marked by unfavorably susceptible responses are at a high gamble of encountering extreme and serious hypersensitive responses.

The majority of the undesirable side effects that have ever been experienced by Acxion users are outlined in this list. You can reduce the number of side effects caused by these pills by following your doctor's instructions and not increasing or decreasing the interval between doses.

Serious Incidental effects

Acxion weight reduction pills have a few serious incidental effects which can cause heart and lung issues.

Obscured vision

Chest torment

Diminished capacity to work out

Trouble relaxing

Blacking out

Seizure

Serious migraine

Slurred discourse

Enlarging

Shortcoming of body

Inconsistencies while Taking Acxion

Very much like all pills, it is essential to know about the safeguards and inconsistencies related with Acxion Fentermina and its dynamic fixing, phentermine.

The following patients should not take Acxion pills:

In the event that you are diabetic then you can't utilize these pills.

Do not take these pills if you have thyroid disease.

If you are psychotic or have a psychotic disorder that has been diagnosed.

Acxion pills should not be taken by people with glaucoma or serious heart disease who have already had a heart attack.

Patients with hypertension, also known as high blood pressure, should not take these pills.

If you have had a stroke in the past

On the off chance that you have a past or current chronic drug use or reliance issue

If you have a diet pill allergy

Pros and Cons of Acxion:

Your appetite may also be controlled or reduced, and your body fat will be reduced.

If you exercise regularly and eat a nutritious diet, you can lose weight.

Obesity-related health problems can be reduced.

Cons:

These pills might cause serious secondary effects like foggy vision and windedness

You can stifle craving yet weight reduction isn't an assurance simply by taking these pills

You require a medicine from a rehearsing doctor to utilize these pills.

This can only be used by people who are medically obese.

Food cravings return to typical when you quit taking these pills.

Acxion Surveys

Due to ongoing astounding client audits, Acxion is the most famous decision for its viable weight decrease recipe. As a result, some customers express concern about the negative effects of these pills. Acxion pills have received the following reviews from customers:

Mark: Loses 20 Kilograms "These Acxion pills have helped me lose 20 Kilograms. I took these pills for three months, took a break for a month, and then have been taking them every day or alternate days for the last two months. Micheal – Highly Effective "I have lost 15 kg with Acxion pills. It truly has amazing results." TobyLauren – 10 kgs "I have been using this brand of Mexican phentermine for the last 10 days, and the appetite suppressant and craving suppressant have been great. It has miraculous results as these pills have changed my entire appearance." In just two weeks, I've lost 10 kilograms.

Where can Acxion pills are purchased?

Because Acxion is a Mexican brand, the majority of Mexican pharmacies sell these pills. A legitimate specialist's remedy is an unquestionable requirement on the off chance that you want to purchase these pills. You likewise can look on the web and request these pills by giving a remedy. For the best price, you need to go to Acxion's official website.

Since weight has turned into a pandemic since it influences all age gatherings and is a really general wellbeing concern everywhere. With anorexic pills like Acxion, overweight people might assist with checking their caloric admission to get thinner.

The anorexigenic Acxion pills do not directly aid in weight loss in obese individuals. Additionally, it reduces food intake by controlling your central nervous system and suppressing appetite. For the desired weight loss, you can use these pills in conjunction with a healthy diet and exercise.

Acxion pills are not long-term medications that cannot be overdosed within a certain period of time. On the other hand, in order to observe any weight loss while taking Acxion pills, you are encouraged to follow a healthy diet and engage in daily exercise. Acxion diet pills should not be used if your body measure index is less than 30, as doing so could result in serious side effects.

To ensure your safety and survival, your body stores calories as fat. Working out in the fat-burning zone, spot reduction, and foods or supplements that supposedly make you burn more fat are just a few of the many tricks that claim to increase fat burning.

Instead of looking for a quick fix that is unlikely to work, learn how to burn fat through a variety of forms of exercise if you want to reduce the amount of fat stored in your body. What you need to know is as follows:

How to Burn Fat Consistently Engage in a combination of high, medium, and low-intensity cardiovascular exercise Lift challenging weights, try circuit training, and include compound exercises. Keep an eye on your stress levels. Get enough sleep. Increase your total daily energy expenditure. Eat the right amount of calories to reach your goal. Basics of Burning Fat knowing how your body uses calories for fuel can help you manage your weight. Fat, carbohydrates, and protein provide energy. Which one your body draws from for energy relies upon the sort of movement you're doing.

The majority of people want to use fat for energy. It might appear that the body will store less fat the more fat it can use as fuel. Be that as it may, utilizing fatter doesn't naturally prompt losing more fat. Understanding the most effective way to consume fat beginnings for certain fundamental realities about how your body gets its energy.1

The body essentially involves fat and sugars for fuel. The proportion of which energizes are used will move contingent upon your action. A limited quantity of protein is utilized during exercise, however fixing the muscles after exercise is basically utilized.

Fast-paced running and other high-intensity workouts force the body to use carbs as fuel. The metabolic pathways that can be used to break down carbohydrates for energy are more effective than those that can be used to break down fat. For prolonged, sluggish exercise, fat is used more for energy than carbohydrates.

This is a clear and concise look at energy with a strong takeaway. Using fat as an energy source is less important than burning more calories. Overall, you'll burn more calories the harder you work.

When it comes to losing weight, the kind of fuel you use doesn't matter. What makes a difference is the number of calories you that consume.

Think about it this way: you're most likely to burn fat when you sit or sleep. But you probably don't think that spending more time sitting and sleeping will help you lose weight. The bottom line is that you are not burning more calories just because you are using more fat as an energy source.

Myth of the Fat Burning Zone The basic premise of the theory of the fat burning zone is that working out at a certain heart rate (between 55% and 65% of your maximum heart rate) will allow your body to burn more fat. This is the idea behind the fat burning zone.

Throughout the long term, this hypothesis has become so imbued as far as we can tell that we see it promoted in books, outlines, sites, magazines, and, surprisingly, on cardio machines at the rec center. The difficulty is that it's deceptive.

While working out at lower intensities can be beneficial, it will not necessarily result in a greater loss of body fat. Increasing your exercise intensity is one way to burn more calories.

If you want to burn fatter, this does not necessarily mean that you should avoid low-intensity exercise. You can do specific things to burn more fat, and the most important factor is how often and how long you exercise.

Burn Fat by Combining Cardio You might be unsure of how hard you should work during cardio. You might even believe that vigorous exercise is the only option. All things considered, you can consume more calories and you don't need to invest as much energy making it happens.

But having a variety of activities can help you stimulate all of your energy systems, prevent injuries from overuse, and make your workouts more enjoyable. You can set up a cardio program that incorporates a wide range of activities at various powers.

High-Intensity Cardio For the purposes of this article, high-intensity cardio is exercise that takes place between 80% and 90% of your maximum heart rate. Or, on a 10-point perceived exertion scale, somewhere between a six and an eight if you are not using heart rate zones. This means exercising at a level that makes you feel challenged and leaves you breathless enough to speak in complete sentences.

However, you are not sprinting as fast as you possibly can. High-intensity training can, without a doubt, help people lose weight while also increasing their endurance and aerobic capacity.

You can get similar advantage from short exercises spread over the course of the day as you do with nonstop exercises. For instance, if a 150-pound person ran at 6 mph for 30 minutes, they would burn about 341 calories. On the other hand, if they walked at 3.5 mph for the same amount of time, they would burn 136 calories.

However, the number of calories burned is only one aspect of the equation. Such a large number of extreme focus exercises consistently can seriously jeopardize you in various ways.

Potential Dangers If you exercise too much at high intensity, you put yourself at risk of

Burnout

Developing to can't stand work out

Conflicting exercises

Overtraining

Abuse wounds

In the event that you don't have a lot of involvement in work out, you might not have the molding or the craving for short of breath and testing exercises. In the event that you have any ailment or injury, check with a medical care supplier prior to preparing.

Assuming that you're completing a few days of cardio every week, you would presumably believe only a couple of exercises should fall into the extreme focus range. You can utilize different exercises to target different wellness regions (like perseverance) and permit your body to recuperate. Here are a few instances of how to consolidate extreme focus exercises.

Fast-paced exercise is one way to incorporate high-intensity workouts. For a 20-minute workout that moves quickly, you can use any activity or machine, but the goal is to stay in the high-intensity work zone the entire time. The usual recommendation is twenty minutes, and the majority of people wouldn't want to stay much longer than that.

Tabata preparing is one more type of extreme cardio exercise in which you buckle down for 20 seconds, rest for 10 seconds, and rehash for 4 minutes. You should be out of breath and unable to speak during this workout.

Additionally, high-intensity training can be incorporated through interval training without having to do so continuously. Substitute a hard fragment (e.g., running at a high speed for 30 to 60 seconds) with a recuperation portion (e.g., strolling for 1 to 2 minutes). For the duration of the workout, which typically lasts between 20 and 30 minutes, repeat this series.

Cardio of a Moderate Intensity There are a number of different ways to define moderate-intensity exercise, but it typically ranges from 70 to 80 percent of your maximum heart rate. On a 10-point scale of perceived exertion, that corresponds to levels four through six. You are breathing harder than usual, but you are still able to talk to people without too much trouble5. Instead of trying to fit exercise in whenever you can, plan your day around it. Focusing on your exercise builds the possibilities that you will achieve your objective. The American School of Sports Medication (ACSM) frequently suggests this degree of force in its activity rules. The fat-burning zone typically occupies the lower end of this range.

Moderate-power exercises additionally have a few extraordinary advantages. For instance, even the smallest amount of movement can improve your health while lowering your risk of diabetes, high blood pressure, and heart disease. In addition, it takes time to develop the endurance and strength to perform difficult exercises. You can work at a pace that is more comfortable for you during moderate workouts, allowing you to be more consistent with your program.

Additionally, there are a variety of activities that can typically get you into the moderate heart rate zones. If you work hard enough, even shoveling snow or raking leaves can fall into that category.

Examples of Exercises with a Moderate Intensity For weight loss, the majority of your cardio workouts should probably be of a moderate intensity. A few models include:

A 30-to 45-minute cardio machine exercise

An energetic walk

Riding a bicycle at a medium speed

Low-Force Action

Low-force practice is underneath 60% to 70% of your MHR, or about a level three to five on a 10-point apparent effort scale. One of the most comfortable areas of exercise is without a doubt this level of intensity, which keeps you moving at a pace that is neither too taxing nor too difficult.

Low-intensity exercise is popular due to this fact and the idea that it burns fatter. However, yet, as we've picked up, working at different powers is great for weight loss. That doesn't imply that low-force practice has no reason.

It includes the long, slow exercises you feel like you could do day in and day out. Even better, it includes routines that you already enjoy, like walking, gardening, biking, or gentle stretching.

By doing an extra lap while shopping, taking the stairs, parking farther from the entrance, and performing more physical tasks around the house, you can engage in low-intensity cardio throughout the day. Yoga and Pilates, for example, are low-intensity workouts that support core strength, flexibility, and balance. They can be a part of a routine that is well-rounded.

Consistent exercise's significance It may appear obvious that regular exercise can aid in fat loss. However, it's not just about how many calories you burn. It also involves the changes your body makes when you exercise frequently. You can burn fatter without even trying thanks to many of these adaptations.

The following are some of the advantages of regular exercise.

Improve your effectiveness: Your body turns out to be more effective at conveying and separating oxygen. Simply put, this makes it easier for your cells to burn fat.

Improve your circulation: Because of this, fatty acids can get into the muscle and through the blood more quickly. That implies fat is all the more promptly accessible for energizing the body.

Increment the number and size of mitochondria: These are the power plants in your cells that generate energy within each cell.

Lift Weights to Burn Fat Adding muscle by lifting weights and doing other resistance exercises can also help burn fat. Although many people focus more on cardio to lose weight, strength training is essential to any weight loss plan. Some advantages of weight training are listed below.

Burn Calories: You can increase your afterburn, or the number of calories burned after a workout, by lifting weights at a higher intensity. This indicates that while you exercise, you burn calories, but your body burns calories even after your workout as it returns to its resting state.

Push Digestion Along

An eating routine just way to deal with weight reduction could bring down an individual's resting metabolic rate by up to 20% per day. Even if you cut calories, lifting weights and maintaining muscle helps keep the metabolisms going.

Maintain Muscle Mass If you cut back on calories, you run the risk of losing muscle. Because muscle is a metabolically active organ, losing it results in a loss of the extra calories burned by muscles.

To begin, pick a fundamental all out body exercise and do that about two times per week, with something like one in the middle between. You can do more exercises, increase the intensity, or add more days of strength training as you get stronger. You'll eventually notice and feel a difference in your body, even if it takes a few weeks.

Systems

To consume more fat while strength preparing, here are a few systems that you can use.

Integrate high-intensity aerobics: Aerobics is an incredible method for consuming more calories by joining extreme focus cardio alongside strength preparing works out. When you focus on both cardio and strength in the same workout, you keep your heart rate high by moving from one exercise to another with little to no rest.

Lift significant burdens: On the off chance that you're a fledgling, you ought to move gradually up to significant burdens over the long run. Lifting a lot of weight forces your body to build more lean muscle tissue to handle the extra load once it is ready for it.

Utilize compound motions: Squats, lunges, deadlifts, triceps dips, and other movements that work more than one muscle group can help you lift more weight and burn more calories while also training the body in a functional way.

Try a four-week slow build program for a more structured program that allows you to gradually increase the intensity of cardio and strength workouts.

Running for Weight Loss

The best strategy for losing weight is to combine healthy eating with exercise. Running is a great way to exercise that also helps you lose weight. With a good running program, you can expect to burn calories and excess fat. There are a couple of different elements that will decide your degree of progress on a running get-healthy plan, including knowing the right preparation schedule.

How to Run to Lose Weight Losing weight necessitates a significant calorie deficit. Most specialists suggest that you go for a week by week calorie deficiency of 3,500 to 7,000 calories to shed 1-2 pounds each week.

You can achieve this deficit by either eating fewer calories or exercising more, like running. To achieve your goal, you can also combine the two approaches.

A weight loss rate of one to two pounds per week is safe and acceptable. On the off chance that you are running reliably and adding strength preparing you might be shedding pounds, yet you're presumably likewise acquiring muscle simultaneously.

Your body is getting fitter, stronger, and leaner as a result, but the scale may show a change. In fact, you might even notice an increase in weight at times. Think about using a different approach to keep track of your progress. Observe the difference in how your clothes fit or measure your body fat percentage.

The Importance of a Healthy Diet

Although runners have particular dietary requirements, the fundamental principles of healthy eating remain applicable. Try consuming more whole grains, proteins, and whole fruits and vegetables in addition to larger portions of foods that are high in fat and calories.

Overcompensating for the calories burned by consuming more food and beverages is a common eating error among runners. Despite their regular training, some runners even find that they gain weight or hit a weight loss plateau.

The initial step to hitting your objective is realizing exactly the amount you're eating. Find out how many calories you need to lose weight by using this calculator.

After you run, pay attention to what you eat. Refueling after practice is significant, yet the way that you refuel is critical assuming your objective is weight reduction. The actual demonstration of activity will expand your craving as your body requests more calories to keep it running. If you don't watch out and eat a lot of some unacceptable food varieties, you might wind up surpassing your energy requests.

The theory is that you can reduce muscle soreness by eating soon after a long run or intense workout because studies show that muscles are most receptive to rebuilding glycogen stores.

After your run, opt for a portion-controlled snack like a post-run smoothie or chocolate milk with a banana and yogurt. Focus on protein- and fiber-rich foods at mealtime to keep you full and satisfied.

Sustenance Ways to run for Weight reduction

Here are more tips to keep your eating regimen on target include:

Eat less often: Instead of eating three big meals, break up your calories into five or six smaller ones. This can help keep your metabolism and energy levels in check and stop you from feeling hungry so much that you eat too much.

Keep an eye on the calories in liquids: Even if you run a lot, you don't have to drink sports drinks all the time to stay hydrated. The same is true for soda, coffee drinks, and fruit juices. To maintain adequate hydration, simply drink water.

Reduce carbs: On a 2,000-calorie diet, the typical adult should consume between 225 and 325 grams of carbohydrates per day, or 45 and 65 percent of their daily calories. Assuming you are surpassing this — or are inside the reach yet are as yet incapable to get thinner — trim the carbs somewhat and supplant with lean protein.

Maintain a food diary: One method for forestalling gorging or thoughtless eating is to compose all that you're eating in a diary for half a month. You can see where your diet needs to be improved by reviewing a food diary.

Calories Burned While Running

Running is an efficient and quick way to burn calories. The length of time you run, your pace, and your body size all affect how many calories you burn. However, many runners of average size estimate that they burn approximately 100 calories per mile as a general rule.

According to data from the National Weight Control Registry, planned exercise burns about 2,800 calories per week for people who lose weight and keep it off. Accepting a normal of 100 calories for every mile, that is around 28 miles each week.

It means quite a bit to take note of that this is more than the normal sprinter finishes in a week and is particularly a great deal for another sprinter out of the entryways. Due to the risk of injury, you should gradually increase your mileage until it suits you.

It is possible to achieve your weight loss goal if running is your only form of exercise. Focus only on completing the miles on a weekly schedule and don't worry about your pace or intensity.

Schedule your runs ahead of time, just like you would any other important event. Running eventually helps you burn the calories you need to lose weight.

Running Workouts for Weight Loss The length of time it takes to lose weight can be affected by the kind of running workouts you do. Although there is no "best" running workout, combining different types of training can help you lose the most weight.

Consistency is critical to any fruitful get-healthy plan, particularly one that includes running. Running is a strenuous activity. For some, running every day or even every other day might be too strenuous. However, you won't see the benefits if you only exercise occasionally.

Try running alongside weight training, rowing, cycling, hiking, and other activities. Attempt to do an actual work on most days of the seven day stretch of some sort. The American College of Sports Medicine says that people who lose the most weight do 250 to 300 minutes of moderate exercise a week.3 High-Intensity vs. Low-Intensity Running Workouts When you exercise, your body's use of carbs and fat for fuel can change depending on how fast you go, how long you do it for, and how intense it is. Consider it this way:

Running at high intensities: Because they are a quick energy source, the body relies more on carbs. They give your body the eruption of energy it needs while sending off something like a run. It is similar to lighting a match on paper: It starts to burn hotter and faster, but it ends quickly.

Runs of a lower intensity: Your body gradually switches from carbs to fat during these longer, lower-intensity runs. Fats are more sustainable, even though they are not as immediate a fuel source. Burning fat is more like lighting a candle in this sense: it consumes steadier and longer.

Working out at a steady, slower pace seems reasonable if your goal is to lose weight. Necessarily not. While practicing at a lower force will permit you to consume a more noteworthy extent of calories from fat, working out at a higher power implies that you're consuming more calories in general.

Interval running workouts require you to run at a higher intensity, around 80% or 90% of your maximum heart rate, in order to burn more calories. You are not running a full sprint at this speed, but you are working so hard that you can't talk to anyone.

Begin by doing a 20-minute run at around 80% to 90 percent force. Alternately, you can perform interval training, in which you alternate between workouts of varying intensities. You can make the intervals and repetitions last longer as you progress and get fitter.

Obviously, you shouldn't run going on like this constantly. You need to give your body a chance to recover and rebuild itself after any kind of strenuous activity. A couple of high-intensity runs each week are reasonable.

Complete shorter, longer runs on the other days of the week. You'll be able to run more miles and burn more calories because these runs will feel more consistent. Lastly, hill repeats or indoor treadmill runs can be done to break up boredom and build strength.

Keep in mind that strength training is an important part of your running training. Strength training is a regular part of the routine for runners who lose weight and keep it off. While you are strength training, not only will you burn calories but also your running performance will improve as a result of your increased lean muscle mass. When you run, you'll be able to run faster and for longer and burn more calories.

Even at rest, having lean muscle mass helps you burn more calories throughout the day. Strength preparing likewise forestalls running wounds, so you'll have the option to keep up with your obligation to practice by remaining sans injury.

Every week, try doing weight training or resistance training. Each week, schedule two to three 20- to 30-minute sessions of strength training into your training schedule. To make a difference, you don't have to lift heavy weights. Straightforward body weight activities can be compelling.

Heart Rate to Burn Fat: What It Is and How to Target It If you exercise to lose weight, you've probably been told that you should work in your "fat-burning zone" for the best results. Your fat-consuming zone alludes to the exercise power that gets your body to consume fundamentally fat for fuel and is much of the time estimated utilizing pulse.

The term "fat burning zone" refers to a desired heart rate that necessitates the use of more of your body's stored fat to maintain. A person's VO2 max is typically between 50% and 72% of their fat-burning zone. Even though this zone is referred to as fat-burning, it does not necessarily imply that you will burn more fat than if you exercised at a lower or higher intensity. The fat-burning zone theory ignores the effects of longer workout sessions or more intense exercise.

Your resting heart rate, or RHR, is the number of times your heart beats per minute (BPM) when you are at rest. You can decide this rate by putting your pointer on your wrist or neck and counting the beats you feel for 60 seconds. A sound RHR is generally between 60 to 100 BPM.

Your most extreme pulse (MHR), or the greatest number of times your heart can thump in a moment, is determined by deducting your age from the number 220. Your MHR, for instance, is 190 if you are 30 years old (220 - 30 = 190).

There are various heart-rate zones that correspond to various intensities when it comes to exercise, particularly cardio exercise. The energy systems your body uses during exercise are determined by these levels, which are based on MHR and have a direct impact on how many calories you burn.

Heart Rate for Burning Fat The lowest intensity zone burns fat. Why? Because working at a lower intensity causes the body to use more stored fat (rather than carbs) as its primary fuel source. Some people have misunderstood this to mean that working at a lower intensity makes you burn fatter, but that's not entirely accurate. Actually, hustling will burn more absolute calories — and at last more fat — in less time.3 And it's the quantity of calories you consume by and large that prompts the most weight (and fat) misfortune.

To give you a model, the diagram underneath subtleties both the all-out calories and the fat calories exhausted by a 130-pound lady during cardio work out. When exercising at a higher intensity, the woman burns more total calories and fat calories, as you will see.

This doesn't mean that low-intensity exercise doesn't have a place, especially if you're just starting out and can't keep up with a faster pace.4 if you exercise slower, you might be able to exercise for a lot longer, and that will help you burn more calories and fat.

Along with short, high-intensity interval workouts, endurance exercises should be a staple of a comprehensive fitness program even for more experienced exercisers. While lower-intensity workouts are great for building endurance, you need to work harder during some workouts if you really want to burn fat and lose weight. Interval training, in which you alternate high-intensity exercise with low-intensity recovery periods, is proven to increase fitness and burn more calories than steady-state cardio. Hence, fluctuating exercise power, for example, extreme cardio exercise and consistent state cardio, are significant for a decent work out regime.

Organizing Cardio Exercises

To get in shape, a general cardio timetable would incorporate exercises at different powers inside your objective pulse zone.4 For example, on the off chance that you're doing five cardio exercises seven days, you could have one focused energy exercise, one lower-force exercise, and three some place in the center.

Because you can exercise for longer periods of time with low-intensity cardio, you build more stamina. In turn, this makes you stronger and makes you burn more calories overall.

A novice cardio program allows you gradually to construct perseverance while getting you a bit out of your usual range of familiarity. This way, you won't have to be miserable for the entire workout, but you'll still be pushing yourself and burning more calories. The following is an example program that will assist with kicking you off.

The key is to begin with what you can handle and work your way up gradually. Don't worry too much about how hard you work when you're just getting started. Concentrate more on developing a manageable exercise routine.

Other Considerations Exercise isn't the Only Way to Burn Fat A well-balanced diet, limiting portion sizes, drinking a lot of water, and getting enough sleep can also help you lose weight. The quicker you lose weight, the more options you have.

In addition, cardiovascular exercise is not just about losing weight or burning fat. How to Track Your Weight Loss Progress Have you ever exercised and followed a weight loss diet for several weeks only to see the scale stay at the same number day after day? Regular exercise has been shown to lower your resting heart rate, which in turn lowers your risk of dying early from cardiovascular disease.5 If that is the case, there is a reason why you are not alone. The scale doesn't recount the entire story.

In the event that you're figuring out, your body is changing, as a matter of fact. Your heart is figuring out how to function all the more productively, your course is improving, and somewhere inside your phones, you're really developing more mitochondria.

These progressions are essential for weight reduction to occur, however it's difficult to become amped up for changes that we can't see and feel. So, how can you tell if you're making progress if you can't measure the changes and the scale isn't moving?

How to Keep Track of Your Body Fat

The scale weight is a useful number, but knowing your body fat percentage is even better. Due to the fact that scale weight does not always convey the entire picture, this is crucial. Even though a bodybuilder has a very low body fat percentage, knowing your body fat percentage can give you a better idea of how much fat you really need to lose and, even better, whether you're making progress in your program—things that your scale can't tell you. A bodybuilder will have a lot more muscle than is typical for his weight, so standard height-to-weight measurements like the body mass index (BMI) may place him in the overweight category. Even if you are slimming down and gaining muscle, it is possible for your scale weight to remain the same.

Weight Record (BMI) is a dated, one-sided measure that doesn't represent a few elements, like body structure, nationality, race, orientation, and age.

Regardless of being an imperfect measure, BMI is broadly involved today in the clinical local area since it is an economical and fast strategy for dissecting potential wellbeing status and results.

Bioelectrical impedance scales, calipers, DEXA (dual energy X-ray absorptiometry), hydrostatic weighing, and online calculators like the one below are all available for body fat testing.

Capitalize on your muscle versus fat estimation by:

Examining it once or twice per week. You may not notice those small changes if you measure every day because body fat does not disappear overnight.

Having a similar individual measure you each time. You should stick with the same trainer each time because different trainers will measure you in different ways. Make sure the trainer is very experienced at measuring body fat.

- Using a calendar or journal to keep track of your numbers. Responsibility is vital.
- Taking measurements under constant conditions. When measuring with a bioelectrical impedance scale, always measure under the same conditions. Body fat measurements can be influenced by hydration, food intake, and skin temperature.

The Issue with Scales

Scales don't necessarily in every case give you the entire tale about your body or your weight reduction progress. As a result, using scales on their own is not the best way to monitor your internal health. Although these scales only provide you with an estimate, you might want to consider upgrading to a smart scale that also measures things like body fat percentage, BMI, and muscle mass.

The emotional aspect of weighing oneself is yet another reason why people dislike scales. The issue with bodyweight scales is that they measure everything, including fat, muscle, bones, organs, and even that sip of water or bite of food you've had. This means that stepping on a scale doesn't just give you a number; it can also determine how you feel about yourself and affect your body image.3 When we say weight, we really mean fat, and the scale can't tell you what you've lost or gained, which is important information if you're trying to lose weight.

Why Your Weight Changes The numbers you see on the scale can be different for a variety of reasons. When keeping track of how far you've come in losing weight, it's critical to take into account all of these factors.

Food Weight Gain

Gauging yourself after a feast isn't the smartest thought essentially on the grounds that food adds weight. Your body will also gain that weight when you eat it. It does not imply that you have put on weight; rather, it simply indicates that something has been added to your body (something that will be absorbed through digestion over the following several hours).

Muscle Gain Muscle is denser than fat and takes up less space, so even if you're losing weight, adding muscle could make you weigh more.4

However, that doesn't mean the scale is pointless. As a matter of fact, it's a superb device when you consolidate it with your muscle to fat ratio. If you know these two numbers, you can tell if you're losing the right amount of weight: fat.

Water Weight Gain

Since the body is around 60% water, vacillations in your hydration levels can change the number on a scale. Your body may actually retain water, causing your weight to rise if you are dehydrated or have eaten too much salt. Also, numerous ladies hold water during monthly cycles, which is something else that can roll out that number improvement.

Multiply your weight by your body fat percentage to determine your lean and fat percentages. For instance, an individual who weighs 150 lbs with

21% muscle versus fat has 31 lbs of fat and 118 lbs of lean tissue (150 x 0.21 = 31.5 lbs of fat, 150 - 31.5 = 118 lean tissue).

You will be able to see what you are gaining or losing by keeping track of these numbers on a weekly or monthly basis. Try these strategies to make weighing yourself more beneficial and enjoyable:

To give your body time to adjust to your weight loss program, limit your monthly weigh-ins to once per day or once per week. The scale will not reflect little changes occurring in your body structure.

Keep in mind that the scale counts everything. You are still progressing, even if your scale weight has not changed.

Use scale weight, alongside muscle to fat ratio, for a more exact perspective on your advancement

Weigh first thing, before you eat or drink anything.

Measurements are your best option if the scale freaks you out and you can't do a body fat test.

Instructions to Take Your Body Estimations

Taking body estimations is an extraordinary choice for following advancement since it requires no extravagant hardware and anybody can make it happen. Taking measurements of specific areas can give you an idea of where you're losing fat, which is important because everyone loses fat in different places and in different order. Taking your measurements can reassure you that things are happening—even if you aren't losing fat exactly where you want them to right now.

Start by measuring in clothes that fit tightly (or in no clothes at all) and taking a note of what you're wearing so you can remember to measure in the same clothes the next time. How to go about it:

Bust: Take measurements all the way around the chest, right at the nipple line, but don't pull too hard on the tape.

Calves: Measure all the way around each calf's largest part.

Chest: Just below your bust, measure.

Forearm: The largest part of the arm, just below the elbow, should be measured.

Hips: Place the tape measure in the area of your hips that is the largest.

Thighs: Measure around the greatest piece of every thigh.

Arm up top: Measure the circumference of each arm just above the elbow.

Waist: Take a measurement that is half an inch higher than your belly button or at the tiniest part of your waist.

This progress chart can be used to keep track of your measurements. Take them again one time each week or when a month to check whether you're losing inches.

Don't overlook one of the simplest ways to track progress—how your clothes fit—despite the fact that it may seem obvious. In your weight loss journal, you might want to take a picture of yourself in a bathing suit. If you take a new picture of yourself every month, you'll be surprised at how many changes you notice there as opposed to just looking in the mirror.

You can likewise utilize your garments to monitor your progress.6 Pick one sets of jeans that are somewhat close and give them a shot at regular intervals to perceive how they fit. Take note of how you feel while wearing them and where they feel loose or tight.

If you're looking for a workout for women to lose weight, you probably already know that not everyone loses weight the same way. It may take longer to achieve your goals than it does for others, depending on your fitness level, age, lifestyle, and medical history. For example, there's a general generalization that ladies will quite often get thinner more leisurely than men.

There are a number of factors that contribute to this slower rate of weight loss, such as differences in muscle mass and hormonal differences between the sexes.1 However, it is possible to overcome obstacles that are stifling your progress. You can begin to see the results you want with the right training plan and a positive attitude.

Diet and physical activity both contribute to weight loss. The majority of experts concur that diet has a greater impact on weight loss than exercise alone. However, in addition to reducing calories, exercise has a number of other weight-loss benefits, such as lowering blood pressure, increasing insulin sensitivity, and lowering cholesterol.23 Exercise also releases endorphins, which make losing weight enjoyable and prevent exhaustion. Building muscle, adaptability, and perseverance through exercise can help your self-perception and work on your possibilities supporting weight reduction over the long term.4

It might shock you; yet setting weight reduction to the side and zeroing in on different objectives can assist you with losing more weight. In the event that you end up fixated on weight reduction, address a medical services supplier.

When people are trying to lose weight, the first thing that comes to mind is cardio, or aerobic exercise. Although cardio isn't always the best option and should be done in conjunction with resistance training, it has a number of health benefits and can help you lose weight. Here are a few sorts of cardio to consider.

Strolling

Strolling ought not to be underestimated during weight reduction endeavors. Walking not only aids in maintaining a healthy energy balance, but it is also long-lasting, low-impact, doesn't require recovery time, and helps alleviate stress. Adjusting pressure during weight reduction is urgent. Your body can't tell the difference between physical and other kinds of stress.

It can put a lot of stress on your body to eat less and exercise more frequently in order to lose weight. This can prompt expanded wounds, sicknesses, and burnout, putting forth your weight reduction attempts more testing to stick to.5

Rather than zeroing in on additional serious types of activity, continue to stroll as the mainstay of your activity routine.6 Plan to expand your means every week, or work in more day to day development by taking movement parts from work. High-Intensity Training High-intensity training has its place, but it must be balanced with proper nutrition, rest, and other forms of activity. Daily movement are essential for healthy weight balance. You can complete these workouts even if you don't have much time because they are shorter. One of the best ways to improve your fitness during any workout is through interval training. Work hard for 30 to 60 seconds, take a break, and then do it again. Simply remember that HIIT isn't possible consistently and is exceptionally burdening on your body.

Regular interval training is elevated to the next level through high-intensity exercises in high-intensity interval training (HIIT). Sprint interval training is an example of HIIT, which has been shown to help with diabetes and cardiovascular disease.8 It can also help you improve your body composition effectively and efficiently.

Tabata preparing is one more type of extreme cardio exercise that includes pushing hard for exceptionally brief periods, assisting you with consuming calories and fire up your digestion. Try the Tabata Cardio Workout with a lot of force or the Tabata Low Impact Challenge.

Avoiding Cardio Mistakes: Excessive cardio: Dull movements in cardio works out (like running) increment the gamble of injury and overtraining.10 Change around your everyday practice and go home for the days to recuperate between exercises on a case by case basis.

Adhering to low-power cardio: It's possible that doing cardio in your "fat-burning zone" won't help you lose weight. You will have an advantage in weight loss if you incorporate workouts with a higher intensity.

Weight Training for Women Weight training can improve body composition in both men and women, especially when combined with good nutrition.12 In addition to building stronger muscles, weight lifting aids in energy balance (calorie burning) in a few ways.

To start with, bulk is metabolically dynamic, meaning it consumes calories even very still, not at all like fat tissue which doesn't consume calories. Second, as your body repairs tissues during and after your workout, resistance training makes you burn calories.

If you don't like typical cardiovascular exercise, resistance training alone, combined with a supportive diet, can lead to weight loss. Keep in mind that resistance training efforts will also give your heart and lungs a workout. Research shows that weight loss interventions incorporating resistance training and a calorie deficit are the most effective for reducing body fat percentage. You don't have to swim, run, or cycle to improve your cardiovascular fitness.

More grounded muscles additionally assist with building more grounded bones and lift digestion. If you get bored easily with weight training, circuit training is a fun way to sneak in a resistance workout. This will help you maintain an active lifestyle for years to come and prevent some weight gain and chronic diseases that are typically associated with aging.4 When you do circuit training, you don't take any breaks between exercises, usually combining cardio and strength training. Although circuit training won't likely help you gain strength or muscle mass, it can help you lose weight while maintaining muscle mass and improve your cardiovascular fitness. If this appeals to you, try to incorporate circuit training one to two times per week, or you can supplement your regular strength training routine with circuit training once per week. Maintaining muscle mass is essential during weight loss to prevent regain and maintain optimal metabolism. Make sure to rest your muscles between workouts.

Through simple, focused movements, strength training workouts build muscle. Do a split routine for your upper and lower body or do a total body workout twice a week.

Kettle bell exercises are just as effective at building strength as traditional dumbbell exercises. Resistance bands are an additional option. Simply ensure that you are lifting sufficient weight. Legitimate structure is fundamental for successful and safe strength preparing. In the event that you don't know how to get everything rolling, enroll the assistance of a certified fitness coach.

Monday: 15 minutes of HIIT, with 30 seconds of sprinting and 1 minute of walking alternated every 30 seconds. Perform the Total Body Dumbbell Workout as a follow-up.

Tuesday: 30 to 60 minutes of moderate cardiovascular exercise, like the Cardio Endurance Workout.

Wednesday: Walking, active rest, and mobility training on Thursday: Repeat the dumbbell workout for the entire body.

Friday: HIIT training or cardio at rest; center work

Saturday: Walking and dumbbells for the whole body on Sunday: Walking, active rest, and mobility training Walking and resting are necessary parts of any workout program. Give yourself an extra day off and return tomorrow if you become too tired or sore.

How to Burn Fat Your body stores calories as fat to keep you safe and alive. Working out in the fat-burning zone, spot reduction, and foods or supplements that supposedly make you burn fatter are just a few of the many tricks that claim to increase fat burning.

Instead of looking for a quick fix that is unlikely to work, learn how to burn fat through a variety of forms of exercise if you want to reduce the amount of fat stored in your body. What you need to know is as follows:

Basics of Fat Burning If you want to reduce the amount of fat stored in your body, knowing how your body uses calories as fuel can help you control your weight. Fat, carbohydrates, and protein provide energy. Which one your body draws from for energy relies upon the sort of movement you're doing.

The majority of people want to use fat for energy. It might appear that the body will store less fat the more fat it can use as fuel. Be that as it may, utilizing fatter doesn't naturally prompt losing more fat. Understanding the most effective way to consume fat beginnings for certain fundamental realities about how your body gets its energy.1

The body essentially involves fat and sugars for fuel. The proportion of which energizes are used will move contingent upon your action. A limited quantity of protein is utilized during exercise, however fixing the muscles after exercise is basically utilized.

Fast-paced running and other high-intensity workouts force the body to use carbs as fuel. The metabolic pathways that can be used to break down carbohydrates for energy are more effective than those that can be used to break down fat. For prolonged, sluggish exercise, fat is used more for energy than carbohydrates.

This is a clear and concise look at energy with a strong takeaway. Using fat as an energy source is less important than burning more calories. Overall, you'll burn more calories the harder you work.

When it comes to losing weight, the kind of fuel you use doesn't matter. What makes a difference is the number of calories you that consume.

Think about it this way: you're most likely to burn fat when you sit or sleep. But you probably don't think that spending more time sitting and sleeping will help you lose weight. The bottom line is that you are not burning more calories just because you are using more fat as an energy source.

Myth of the Fat Burning Zone The basic premise of the theory of the fat burning zone is that working out at a certain heart rate (between 55% and 65% of your maximum heart rate) will allow your body to burn more fat. This is the idea behind the fat burning zone.

Throughout the long term, this hypothesis has become so imbued as far as we can tell that we see it promoted in books, outlines, sites, magazines, and, surprisingly, on cardio machines at the rec center. The difficulty is that it's deceptive.

While working out at lower intensities can be beneficial, it will not necessarily result in a greater loss of body fat. Increasing your exercise intensity is one way to burn more calories.

If you want to burn fatter, this does not necessarily mean that you should avoid low-intensity exercise. You can do specific things to burn more fat, and the most important factor is how often and how long you exercise.

Burn Fat by Combining Cardio You might be unsure of how hard you should work during cardio. You might even believe that vigorous exercise is the only option. All things considered, you can consume more calories and you don't need to invest as much energy making it happens.

But having a variety of activities can help you stimulate all of your energy systems, prevent injuries from overuse, and make your workouts more enjoyable. You can set up a cardio program that incorporates a wide range of activities at various powers.

High-Intensity Cardio For the purposes of this article, high-intensity cardio is exercise that takes place between 80% and 90% of your maximum heart rate. Or, on a 10-point perceived exertion scale, somewhere between a six and an eight if you are not using heart rate zones. This means exercising at a level that makes you feel challenged and leaves you breathless enough to speak in complete sentences.

However, you are not sprinting as fast as you possibly can. High-intensity training can, without a doubt, help people lose weight while also increasing their endurance and aerobic capacity.

You can get similar advantage from short exercises spread over the course of the day as you do with nonstop exercises. For instance, if a 150-pound person ran at 6 mph for 30 minutes, they would burn about 341 calories.3 On the other hand, if they walked at 3.5 mph for the same amount of time, they would burn 136 calories.

However, the number of calories burned is only one aspect of the equation. Such a large number of extreme focus exercises consistently can seriously jeopardize you in various ways.

Potential Dangers If you exercise too much at high intensity, you put yourself at risk of

- Burnout

- Developing to can't stand work out
- Conflicting exercises
- Overtraining

Abuse wounds

In the event that you don't have a lot of involvement in work out, you might not have the molding or the craving for short of breath and testing exercises. In the event that you have any ailment or injury, check with a medical care supplier prior to preparing.

Assuming that you're completing a few days of cardio every week, you would presumably believe only a couple of exercises should fall into the extreme focus range. You can utilize different exercises to target different wellness regions (like perseverance) and permit your body to recuperate. Here are a few instances of how to consolidate extreme focus exercises.

Fast-paced exercise is one way to incorporate high-intensity workouts. For a 20-minute workout that moves quickly, you can use any activity or machine, but the goal is to stay in the high-intensity work zone the entire time. The usual recommendation is twenty minutes, and the majority of people wouldn't want to stay much longer than that.

Tabata preparing is one more type of extreme cardio exercise in which you buckle down for 20 seconds, rest for 10 seconds, and rehash for 4 minutes. You should be out of breath and unable to speak during this workout.

Additionally, high-intensity training can be incorporated through interval training without having to do so continuously. Substitute a hard fragment (e.g., running at a high speed for 30 to 60 seconds) with a recuperation portion (e.g., strolling for 1 to 2 minutes). For the duration of the workout, which typically lasts between 20 and 30 minutes, repeat this series.

Cardio of a Moderate Intensity There are a number of different ways to define moderate-intensity exercise, but it typically ranges from 70 to 80 percent of your maximum heart rate. On a 10-point scale of perceived exertion, that corresponds to levels four through six. You are breathing harder than usual, but you are still able to talk to people without too much trouble5. Instead of trying to fit exercise in whenever you can, plan your day around it. Focusing on your exercise builds the possibilities that you will achieve your objective. The American School of Sports Medication (ACSM) frequently suggests this degree of force in its activity rules. The fat-burning zone typically occupies the lower end of this range.

Moderate-power exercises additionally have a few extraordinary advantages. For instance, even the smallest amount of movement can improve your health while lowering your risk of diabetes, high blood pressure, and heart disease. In addition, it takes time to develop the endurance and strength to perform difficult exercises. You can work at a pace that is more comfortable for you during moderate workouts, allowing you to be more consistent with your program.

Made in United States
Troutdale, OR
04/02/2024

18885445R00050